Yoga for Stress Relief Finding Serenity in a Chaotic World

Williams

Yoga for Stress Relief Finding Serenity in a Chaotic World

Copyright © 2023 by Williams

All rights reserved. No part of this book may be reproduced or transmitted in any form or by any means, electronic or mechanical, including photocopying, recording, or by any information storage and retrieval system, without permission in writing from the publisher.

This book is a work of fiction. Names, characters, places, and incidents either are the product of the author's imagination or are used fictitiously. Any resemblance to actual events, locales, persons, living or dead, is entirely coincidental.

The first edition was published in 2023

ISBN:

Published by:
Ujwal
1663 Liberty Drive
Hyderabad, IN 47403
www.ujwalpublishers.com

This book is self-published using on-demand printing and publishing, which allows it to be printed and distributed globally.

TABLE OF CONTENTS

Chapter 1: Understanding Stress and its Impact on Mental Health 06

The Relationship between Stress and Mental Health

Common Symptoms of Stress

The Toll of Chronic Stress on the Mind and Body

Chapter 2: Introduction to Yoga as a Tool for Stress Relief 12

The Origins and Philosophy of Yoga

How Yoga Supports Mental Health

The Mind-Body Connection in Yoga Practice

Chapter 3: Essential Yoga Techniques for Stress Relief 18

Breathing Exercises (Pranayama) for Calming the Mind

Gentle Yoga Poses for Relaxation and Stress Reduction

Meditation and Mindfulness Practices for Stress Relief

Chapter 4: Creating a Personalized Yoga Practice for Stress Relief   25

Assessing Your Stress Triggers and Needs

Designing a Yoga Routine for Stress Management

Incorporating Yoga into Your Daily Life

Chapter 5: Yoga and Lifestyle Changes for Long-Term Stress Management   31

The Importance of Self-Care in Stress Reduction

Nurturing Healthy Relationships and Boundaries

Finding Balance in Work, Rest, and Play

Chapter 6: Yoga for Specific Stress-Related Conditions   37

Yoga for Anxiety and Panic Disorders

Yoga for Depression and Mood Disorders

Yoga for Insomnia and Sleep Disorders

Chapter 7: Yoga and Beyond Integrating Other Stress-Relieving Practices   43

Ayurveda: The Sister Science of Yoga for Holistic Healing

Nutrition and Diet for Stress Reduction

Exploring Other Complementary Therapies for Stress Relief

Chapter 8: Overcoming Challenges and Maintaining Motivation 49

Overcoming Resistance to Change and Establishing a Routine

Dealing with Setbacks and Managing Expectations

Cultivating Mindfulness and Gratitude for Long-Term Well-Being

Chapter 9: The Power of Community and Support56

Joining Yoga Classes and Finding Like-Minded Individuals

Building a Support Network for Stress Relief

Sharing Your Journey and Inspiring Others

Chapter 10: Embracing Serenity in a Chaotic World 63

Embracing Imperfections and Letting Go of Control

Cultivating Inner Peace and Serenity Through Yoga

Living a Balanced and Stress-Free Life in a Chaotic World

Chapter 1: Understanding Stress and its Impact on Mental Health

The Relationship between Stress and Mental Health

In today's fast-paced and demanding world, stress has become an inevitable part of our lives. Whether it's work pressures, relationship issues, or financial worries, stress can creep into every aspect of our existence and wreak havoc on our mental health. Understanding the relationship between stress and mental health is crucial for anyone seeking to find serenity in this chaotic world. This subchapter aims to shed light on this connection and provide valuable insights for individuals looking to alleviate stress through the practice of yoga.

Stress, when left unmanaged, can have severe repercussions on our mental health. It can trigger anxiety, depression, and even lead to more serious conditions such as post-traumatic stress disorder (PTSD). When our bodies are exposed to chronic stress, the brain releases excessive amounts of cortisol, a stress hormone that can disrupt the normal functioning of our brain cells. This imbalance affects our mood, memory, and overall cognitive abilities, making it even more challenging to deal with stress effectively.

Fortunately, yoga offers a holistic approach to combat stress and preserve mental well-being. By combining physical postures (asanas), breathing techniques (pranayama), and meditation, yoga helps individuals release tension, reduce anxiety, and restore inner balance. Regular practice of yoga not only strengthens the body but also calms the mind, enabling individuals to better cope with stressors in their daily lives.

Yoga promotes mindfulness, a state of being fully present in the moment, without judgment or attachment. Through mindful awareness, individuals can identify stress triggers and develop healthier coping mechanisms. Moreover, yoga encourages deep breathing, which activates the body's relaxation response, counteracting the fight-or-flight response triggered by stress.

By incorporating yoga into their lives, individuals can experience a profound shift in their mental health. They become more resilient, better able to manage stress, and cultivate a sense of serenity amidst chaos. The regular practice of yoga also enhances self-awareness, allowing individuals to recognize when they are becoming overwhelmed and take proactive steps to mitigate stress before it takes a toll on their mental well-being.

In conclusion, the relationship between stress and mental health is undeniable. However, with the powerful tool of yoga, individuals can reclaim their mental serenity in a chaotic world. By practicing yoga regularly and incorporating its principles into their lives, anyone can find relief from stress and nurture their mental health. So, take a deep breath, roll out your yoga mat, and embark on a journey of self-discovery and tranquility.

Common Symptoms of Stress

Stress is something that affects us all at some point in our lives. Whether it's due to work pressures, relationship issues, financial worries, or any other life circumstance, stress can take a toll on our physical, mental, and emotional well-being. In this subchapter, we will explore the common symptoms of stress and how yoga can help alleviate them.

One of the most noticeable symptoms of stress is an increased heart rate. When we're stressed, our bodies release adrenaline, which can cause our heart to race and our blood pressure to rise. This can lead to feelings of anxiety and restlessness, making it difficult to relax and unwind. Yoga, with its focus on deep breathing and relaxation techniques, can help regulate our heart rate and bring a sense of calm to our bodies and minds.

Another common symptom of stress is muscle tension and pain. When we're under stress, our muscles tend to tighten up, leading to headaches, backaches, and overall discomfort. Yoga offers a variety of stretching and strengthening exercises that can help release tension and promote flexibility. By practicing yoga regularly, we can learn to identify areas of tension in our bodies and work on releasing them through gentle stretches and poses.

Stress can also have a negative impact on our sleep patterns. Many people find it difficult to fall asleep or stay asleep when they're stressed. This can lead to fatigue, irritability, and difficulty concentrating during the day. Yoga promotes relaxation and can help improve the quality of our sleep. By incorporating calming breathing exercises and gentle yoga poses into our bedtime routine, we can create a peaceful environment for sleep and enhance our overall well-being.

In addition to these physical symptoms, stress can also affect our mental and emotional health. It can lead to feelings of overwhelm, sadness, and anxiety. Yoga, with its focus on mindfulness and meditation, can help quiet the mind and bring a sense of peace and clarity. By practicing yoga, we can learn to manage our stress levels more effectively and cultivate a greater sense of serenity in our daily lives.

In conclusion, stress is a common experience that can have a significant impact on our well-being. By recognizing the common symptoms of stress and incorporating yoga into our lives, we can find relief and serenity in the midst of a chaotic world. Whether you're a seasoned yogi or new to the practice, exploring the benefits of yoga for stress relief can be a transformative journey towards a more balanced and peaceful life.

The Toll of Chronic Stress on the Mind and Body

In today's fast-paced and chaotic world, stress has become an inevitable part of our lives. It seems like everyone is constantly juggling multiple responsibilities, striving to meet deadlines, and dealing with various pressures. While a certain amount of stress can be beneficial, chronic stress can take a toll on both our minds and bodies. In this subchapter, we will explore the damaging effects of chronic stress and how yoga can provide relief and restore serenity.

When stress becomes a chronic condition, it can wreak havoc on our mental well-being. Anxiety, depression, and mood swings are commonly associated with prolonged stress. The constant state of heightened alertness can lead to a decrease in concentration, memory problems, and difficulty making decisions. Moreover, chronic stress can negatively impact our sleep patterns, causing insomnia or restlessness, further exacerbating our mental distress.

Not only does chronic stress affect our mental health, but it also takes a significant toll on our physical well-being. Prolonged stress weakens our immune system, making us more susceptible to infections and diseases. It can lead to headaches, muscle tension, and even chronic pain conditions like fibromyalgia. Additionally, stress can disturb our digestive system, causing issues such as irritable bowel syndrome and ulcers. Chronic stress can even accelerate the aging process, leading to premature wrinkles and hair loss.

Fortunately, yoga offers a holistic approach to combat chronic stress and its detrimental effects on the mind and body. Through a combination of physical postures (asanas), breathing exercises (pranayama), and meditation, yoga helps to calm the nervous system, reducing stress hormones such as cortisol. Regular practice of yoga promotes relaxation, enhances mental clarity, and improves overall mood.

Moreover, yoga's emphasis on breath awareness and mindful movement helps to release physical tension stored in the body, relieving muscular pain and promoting flexibility. It also aids in improving sleep patterns, allowing for a more restful and rejuvenating experience. By incorporating yoga into our daily routine, we can restore balance, strengthen our resilience, and cultivate serenity amidst the chaos of life.

In conclusion, chronic stress is a pervasive issue that affects both our minds and bodies. It is essential to recognize the damaging effects of stress and take proactive measures to mitigate its impact. Yoga provides a powerful tool for stress relief, offering a comprehensive approach to restore serenity in our lives. By embracing the practice of yoga, we can find solace in the midst of chaos and reclaim our mental and physical well-being.

Chapter 2: Introduction to Yoga as a Tool for Stress Relief

The Origins and Philosophy of Yoga

Yoga, an ancient practice that originated in India thousands of years ago, has gained immense popularity in recent times as a means to find serenity and relief from the chaos of our modern world. This subchapter delves into the fascinating origins and philosophy of yoga, shedding light on the principles that form the foundation of this transformative practice.

The origins of yoga can be traced back to the Indus Valley Civilization, where archaeological findings suggest that yoga was practiced as early as 5000 BCE. However, it was in the classical period of yoga, around 500 BCE, that the philosophy and teachings of yoga were systematized by sage Patanjali in his seminal work, the Yoga Sutras.

At its core, yoga is not merely a physical exercise but a holistic approach to achieving balance and harmony within oneself. The word "yoga" itself comes from the Sanskrit root "yuj," which means to unite or join. This reflects the underlying philosophy of yoga, which aims to unite the mind, body, and spirit, creating a state of inner peace and tranquility.

One of the fundamental principles of yoga is the belief in the interconnectedness of all beings. Yoga teaches us that we are not separate entities but part of a larger whole, intimately connected to the world around us. This philosophy cultivates a sense of compassion, empathy, and kindness towards ourselves and others.

Another key aspect of yoga is the practice of mindfulness and self-awareness. Through various techniques such as breath control (pranayama), physical postures (asanas), and meditation, yoga enables individuals to develop a heightened sense of awareness and presence in the present moment. This helps to alleviate stress, anxiety, and the constant mental chatter that often plagues our minds.

Yoga also emphasizes the importance of self-discipline and self-reflection. It encourages individuals to cultivate positive habits, make conscious choices, and take responsibility for their actions. By developing self-discipline, we can create a sense of inner strength and resilience, enabling us to navigate the challenges of life with grace and composure.

In conclusion, the origins and philosophy of yoga are deeply rooted in ancient wisdom, offering a comprehensive approach to finding serenity and relief from the chaotic world we live in. By embracing the principles of interconnectedness, mindfulness, self-discipline, and self-awareness, yoga empowers individuals to cultivate a deeper sense of peace and well-being. Whether you are a seasoned yogi or new to the practice, exploring the origins and philosophy of yoga can provide valuable insights and guidance on your journey towards finding inner serenity.

How Yoga Supports Mental Health

In today's fast-paced and chaotic world, it is essential to prioritize mental health and find ways to relieve stress. One effective method that has been practiced for centuries is yoga. Yoga is not just a physical exercise; it is a holistic practice that benefits both the body and mind. In this subchapter, we will explore how yoga supports mental health and provides serenity in a world filled with chaos.

Yoga is renowned for its ability to reduce stress and anxiety. The combination of deep breathing, physical postures, and meditation in yoga helps to activate the parasympathetic nervous system, which promotes relaxation and a sense of calm. By practicing yoga regularly, individuals can learn to manage stress better and develop resilience to life's challenges.

Another way yoga supports mental health is by improving sleep quality. As we know, a lack of sleep can lead to increased stress, anxiety, and even depression. Yoga helps to relax the mind and body, preparing it for a restful sleep. Certain yoga poses, such as forward bends and inversions, can stimulate the production of calming hormones, promoting a more peaceful night's sleep.

Yoga also encourages mindfulness, which is a key practice for mental well-being. Mindfulness involves being fully present in the moment and non-judgmentally observing thoughts and sensations. Through yoga, individuals can cultivate mindfulness by focusing on their breath, body sensations, and movement. This practice helps to quiet the mind, reduce negative thinking patterns, and increase self-awareness.

In addition, yoga provides a sense of community and support. Many yoga classes offer a welcoming environment where individuals can connect with like-minded people, share experiences, and build a support network. This sense of belonging can be particularly beneficial for those struggling with mental health issues, as it creates a safe space to express emotions and receive encouragement.

Lastly, yoga promotes self-care and self-compassion. In a world that often prioritizes productivity and achievement, it is crucial to take time for ourselves and nurture our well-being. Yoga encourages individuals to listen to their bodies, honor their limits, and practice self-compassion. By dedicating time to yoga, individuals learn to prioritize self-care and develop a healthier relationship with themselves.

In conclusion, yoga is a powerful practice that supports mental health and provides serenity in a chaotic world. By incorporating yoga into our lives, we can reduce stress, improve sleep quality, cultivate mindfulness, find a supportive community, and prioritize self-care. Whether you are a beginner or an experienced practitioner, exploring the benefits of yoga can have a transformative impact on your mental well-being.

The Mind-Body Connection in Yoga Practice

Yoga is not just a physical exercise; it is a holistic practice that connects the mind and body. In today's chaotic world, finding serenity and stress relief is essential, and yoga offers a path to achieving this balance. In this subchapter, we will explore the profound mind-body connection and how it is cultivated through yoga practice.

Yoga, derived from ancient Indian philosophy, encompasses various techniques that unite the mind, body, and spirit. It involves physical postures (asanas), breath control (pranayama), meditation, and mindfulness. Through these practices, individuals can experience a deep sense of inner peace and harmony.

The mind-body connection in yoga is based on the understanding that our physical and mental well-being are interconnected. Our thoughts, emotions, and stress levels can directly affect our physical health, and vice versa. Yoga helps us tap into this connection and address imbalances in both aspects.

As we move through different asanas, paying attention to our breath and body sensations, we become more aware of our thoughts and emotions. This heightened awareness allows us to observe and let go of negative thoughts and emotions that contribute to stress and anxiety. By releasing these mental burdens, we create space for positive energy and a sense of calm.

Moreover, yoga promotes physical strength, flexibility, and balance. As we challenge our bodies in various poses, we learn to work with our limitations and find acceptance. This acceptance extends beyond the physical realm and permeates into our mental and emotional state. We become more resilient to stressors, finding balance even in the face of chaos.

Through regular yoga practice, individuals learn to cultivate mindfulness, which is the art of being fully present in the moment. This mindfulness extends beyond the yoga mat and becomes a way of life. We become more attuned to our bodies' needs, recognizing when we need rest, nourishment, or self-care.

In conclusion, the mind-body connection in yoga is a transformative aspect of the practice. By uniting our physical and mental states, we can find serenity and relief from the stresses of our chaotic world. Yoga offers a path to inner peace, strength, and balance. Whether you are a seasoned yogi or a beginner, exploring the mind-body connection through yoga can bring profound benefits to your well-being.

Chapter 3: Essential Yoga Techniques for Stress Relief

Breathing Exercises (Pranayama) for Calming the Mind

Introduction:

In the chaotic world we live in, stress has become an integral part of our daily lives. However, there is a solution that has been practiced for centuries - yoga. One of the fundamental aspects of yoga is pranayama, which involves various breathing exercises that can help calm the mind and alleviate stress. In this subchapter, we will explore a range of pranayama techniques that can be easily incorporated into your daily routine, offering you serenity amidst the chaos.

1.   Deep   Belly   Breathing:
Start by sitting in a comfortable position, with your spine straight and relaxed. Place one hand on your belly and the other on your chest. Take a deep breath in through your nose, allowing your belly to rise as you fill your lungs with air. Exhale slowly through your nose, feeling your belly sink. Repeat this cycle for a few minutes, focusing on the sensation of your breath as it enters and leaves your body. This technique helps reduce anxiety and promotes a sense of calmness.

2.   Alternate   Nostril   Breathing:
Sit in a comfortable position and close your right nostril with your thumb. Inhale deeply through your left nostril, then close it with your ring finger. Release your thumb and exhale through your right nostril. Inhale through the right nostril, close it, and exhale

through the left. Repeat this cycle for a few minutes, allowing the rhythmic flow of your breath to balance your mind and body. This technique helps restore equilibrium and reduces mental fatigue.

3.   Box   Breathing: Imagine a box shape in your mind. Inhale deeply through your nose for a count of four, visualizing the first side of the box. Hold your breath for a count of four, visualizing the second side. Exhale slowly through your nose for a count of four, visualizing the third side. Finally, hold your breath for a count of four, visualizing the fourth side. Repeat this cycle for several minutes, allowing the regularity of your breath to bring tranquility to your mind. This technique helps improve focus and concentration.

Conclusion:

Incorporating these breathing exercises into your yoga practice or daily routine can significantly reduce stress levels and promote a sense of serenity. As you embark on this journey of self-discovery through yoga, remember that the power of your breath can be a tool for calming your mind amidst the chaos of life. Take a few moments each day to connect with your breath, and you will discover the transformative effects it can have on your overall well-being.

Gentle Yoga Poses for Relaxation and Stress Reduction

In today's fast-paced and chaotic world, finding moments of serenity and relaxation can seem like an impossible task. But fear not, for the ancient practice of yoga offers a pathway to inner peace and stress relief. This subchapter focuses on gentle yoga poses that are specifically designed to help you unwind, relax, and reduce stress.

Yoga is a holistic approach to wellness that combines physical postures, breathing techniques, and mindfulness to create a harmonious balance between the mind, body, and spirit. The gentle yoga poses discussed here can be practiced by anyone, regardless of age or fitness level, making them accessible to beginners as well as seasoned yogis.

One of the most effective gentle yoga poses for relaxation is the Child's Pose (Balasana). This pose involves sitting on your knees and bending forward, resting your torso on your thighs and your forehead on the mat. This gentle forward fold elongates the spine, releases tension in the neck and shoulders, and promotes a sense of calm and introspection.

Another beneficial pose for stress reduction is the Legs-Up-The-Wall Pose (Viparita Karani). This pose involves lying on your back with your legs extended vertically against a wall. By reversing the effects of gravity, this pose allows for increased blood flow to the brain, which promotes relaxation and relieves anxiety. It also helps to reduce swelling in the legs and feet, making it an excellent choice for those who spend long hours on their feet.

To release tension in the back and shoulders, the Cat-Cow Pose (Marjaryasana-Bitilasana) is highly recommended. This gentle flow involves moving between arching the back like a cat and lifting the chest and tailbone like a cow. It stretches the spine, opens the chest, and helps to alleviate stress and fatigue.

Finally, the Corpse Pose (Savasana) is a must for complete relaxation. This pose involves lying flat on your back with your arms relaxed by your sides and your legs slightly apart. It allows for deep relaxation, rejuvenation, and a welcome break from the constant busyness of the mind.

By incorporating these gentle yoga poses into your daily routine, you can find solace, relaxation, and stress reduction in the midst of a chaotic world. Take a few moments each day to reconnect with yourself, breathe deeply, and let go of the stress and tension that weigh you down. Allow yoga to be your sanctuary, offering a refuge of peace and tranquility in an otherwise hectic life.

Meditation and Mindfulness Practices for Stress Relief

In today's fast-paced and chaotic world, stress has become an inevitable part of our lives. The constant demands from work, relationships, and other responsibilities can leave us feeling overwhelmed and exhausted. However, amidst this chaos, there is a powerful tool that can help restore balance and serenity – meditation and mindfulness practices.

Meditation is an ancient practice that has been used for centuries to quiet the mind and cultivate inner peace. By focusing on the breath or a specific mantra, meditation allows us to let go of racing thoughts and enter a state of deep relaxation. Regular meditation practice has been scientifically proven to reduce stress levels, lower blood pressure, and improve overall well-being.

Mindfulness, on the other hand, is the practice of being fully present in the moment, without judgment or attachment. It involves paying attention to our thoughts, emotions, and physical sensations with curiosity and acceptance. By practicing mindfulness, we can break free from the grip of stress and learn to respond to life's challenges with clarity and calmness.

Incorporating meditation and mindfulness into your yoga practice can greatly enhance its stress-relieving benefits. During yoga, we already focus on the breath and the body's sensations, which naturally helps to quiet the mind. However, by adding specific meditation and mindfulness techniques, we can deepen our practice and experience even greater stress relief.

One powerful technique is the body scan meditation, where you systematically bring your attention to each part of the body, starting from the toes and moving up to the top of the head. This practice not only helps you become more aware of physical tension but also allows you to release it, promoting a deep sense of relaxation.

Another effective mindfulness practice is mindful walking, where you bring your full attention to the act of walking – feeling the ground beneath your feet, noticing the movement of your legs, and being aware of your surroundings. This simple practice can be done anywhere and can help you cultivate a sense of grounding and presence, even during the busiest of days.

By incorporating meditation and mindfulness into your yoga practice, you can create a powerful stress-relieving routine that nourishes both your body and mind. Remember, stress is not something we can completely eliminate from our lives, but with these practices, we can learn to navigate it with grace and find serenity amidst the chaos. So take a deep breath, roll out your yoga mat, and let the journey towards stress relief begin.

Chapter 4: Creating a Personalized Yoga Practice for Stress Relief

Assessing Your Stress Triggers and Needs

In our modern world, stress has become an unavoidable part of life. Whether it's work pressures, financial burdens, or personal relationships, stress can creep into every corner of our existence, leaving us feeling overwhelmed and drained. However, by understanding and addressing the triggers of our stress, we can take proactive steps towards finding serenity in the chaos through the practice of yoga.

Yoga offers a holistic approach to stress relief, providing physical, mental, and emotional support. But before you can fully embrace the healing powers of yoga, it's important to assess your stress triggers and needs. This subchapter will guide you through a self-reflection process to help identify the root causes of your stress and determine what you need to find balance and serenity.

Firstly, it's crucial to become aware of your stress triggers. Take a moment to reflect on the situations, people, or events that tend to evoke a stress response in you. Is it deadlines at work? Conflict with loved ones? Financial worries? By pinpointing these triggers, you can start to understand the specific areas of your life that require attention and nurturing.

Next, consider what you need in order to alleviate stress. Perhaps you require more time for self-care, such as practicing yoga, meditation, or engaging in hobbies that bring you joy. Maybe you need to establish boundaries in your relationships or seek support from a therapist or counselor. Recognizing your needs is the first step towards creating a personalized stress relief plan.

Yoga can play a significant role in addressing your stress triggers and needs. Through the practice of asanas (yoga poses), pranayama (breathing techniques), and meditation, you can cultivate a sense of calm and inner peace. Yoga provides a safe space for self-exploration, allowing you to release tension and pent-up emotions, while also building strength, flexibility, and resilience.

By regularly engaging in yoga for stress relief, you can develop a deeper understanding of yourself and your stress patterns. Over time, you'll become more attuned to your body and mind, noticing the subtle signs of stress before they escalate. This self-awareness empowers you to take proactive steps towards finding serenity in a chaotic world.

Remember, yoga is a journey, and stress relief is not an overnight process. Be patient and gentle with yourself as you navigate through this subchapter and incorporate yoga into your life. By assessing your stress triggers and needs, you're already taking a significant step towards reclaiming your inner peace and finding serenity amidst the chaos.

Designing a Yoga Routine for Stress Management

In today's fast-paced and chaotic world, stress has become an inevitable part of our lives. The constant pressure to meet deadlines, fulfill responsibilities, and juggle multiple tasks can leave us feeling overwhelmed and exhausted. However, there is a powerful tool that can help us find serenity amidst this chaos – yoga.

Yoga is not just a physical exercise; it is a holistic practice that combines physical postures, breath control, meditation, and relaxation techniques. It has been practiced for centuries and is known for its numerous benefits, including stress relief. By incorporating yoga into your daily routine, you can effectively manage stress and find inner peace.

When designing a yoga routine specifically for stress management, it is important to focus on certain aspects. Firstly, choose yoga postures that promote relaxation and release tension from the body. Forward bends, such as Uttanasana (Standing Forward Fold), and gentle backbends, like Bhujangasana (Cobra Pose), can help stretch and soothe the muscles, allowing you to release physical stress.

Breathing exercises, or pranayama, are another essential component of a stress-relieving yoga routine. Techniques like Nadi Shodhana (Alternate Nostril Breathing) and Kapalabhati (Skull Shining Breath) can help calm the mind and reduce anxiety. These practices enhance the flow of oxygen in the body, promoting a sense of calmness and clarity.

Meditation is a powerful tool for stress management. By incorporating meditation into your routine, you can train your mind to focus on the present moment, letting go of worries and anxieties. Start with just a few minutes of seated meditation, gradually increasing the duration as you become more comfortable.

Finally, relaxation techniques, such as Savasana (Corpse Pose), should be included at the end of your yoga routine. This pose allows your body and mind to completely relax, enabling you to experience deep rest and rejuvenation.

Remember, the key to a successful yoga routine for stress management is consistency. Aim to practice yoga at least three to four times a week, gradually increasing the frequency as you progress. Additionally, listen to your body and modify the postures as needed to suit your individual needs and limitations.

In conclusion, designing a yoga routine for stress management can be a transformative experience. By incorporating physical postures, breath control, meditation, and relaxation techniques, you can find serenity in the midst of a chaotic world. Take the first step towards a stress-free life by embracing the practice of yoga.

Incorporating Yoga into Your Daily Life

Yoga has gained immense popularity over the years as a powerful tool for stress relief and finding serenity in a chaotic world. Its ancient practice offers numerous benefits for both the mind and body, making it an essential part of our daily routines. By incorporating yoga into your daily life, you can experience a transformation that goes beyond the mat and into every aspect of your existence.

One of the key aspects of incorporating yoga into your daily life is establishing a regular practice. Consistency is the key to reaping the full benefits of yoga. Whether you choose to practice in the morning to energize your day or in the evening to unwind, finding a time that works best for you is crucial. Carving out just a few minutes each day to dedicate to yoga can make a world of difference in reducing stress and increasing your overall well-being.

Another way to integrate yoga into your daily life is by cultivating mindfulness. Yoga teaches us to be present in the moment, to observe our thoughts and bodily sensations without judgment. By bringing this mindfulness into our daily activities, we can transform mundane tasks into opportunities for self-reflection and inner peace. Whether it's washing dishes, walking in nature, or waiting in line, you can practice deep breathing and bring your awareness to the present moment, allowing stress to melt away.

In addition to practicing on the mat and cultivating mindfulness, incorporating yoga into your daily life also involves adopting a yogic lifestyle. This includes making conscious choices about what you eat, how you move your body, and the thoughts you entertain. Nourishing your body with wholesome, plant-based foods, engaging in regular physical activity, and cultivating positive thoughts and intentions are all integral parts of a yogic lifestyle.

Moreover, incorporating yoga into your daily life extends beyond the individual level. Yoga teaches us the importance of connection and compassion towards others. By practicing kindness, empathy, and non-judgment, we can create a more harmonious and peaceful world. Engaging in community yoga classes, participating in volunteer work, or simply showing kindness to strangers can foster a sense of unity and contribute to the collective well-being.

In conclusion, incorporating yoga into your daily life is a transformative journey that goes beyond physical exercise. By establishing a regular practice, cultivating mindfulness, adopting a yogic lifestyle, and embracing a sense of community, you can experience the profound benefits of yoga in every aspect of your existence. So, take a deep breath, roll out your mat, and embark on a journey towards serenity and stress relief.

Chapter 5: Yoga and Lifestyle Changes for Long-Term Stress Management

The Importance of Self-Care in Stress Reduction

In our fast-paced and chaotic world, stress has become an inevitable part of our daily lives. From demanding work schedules to personal responsibilities, it seems like there is always something that keeps us on our toes. However, amidst all the chaos, it is crucial to prioritize self-care, and yoga can be an excellent tool to achieve stress reduction and find serenity.

Self-care refers to the practice of intentionally taking care of your physical, mental, and emotional well-being. It involves carving out time for activities that nurture and rejuvenate you, ultimately leading to a better quality of life. While it may seem like a luxury or an indulgence, self-care is a necessity, especially when it comes to managing stress.

Yoga, with its mind-body approach, is a powerful practice that promotes self-care and stress reduction. Through a combination of physical postures, breathing exercises, and meditation, yoga helps create a sense of balance and calmness within oneself. It allows individuals to connect with their bodies, quiet their minds, and release tension, ultimately reducing stress levels.

One of the main reasons why self-care is crucial for stress reduction is that it helps to replenish and recharge our energy reserves. When we constantly push ourselves without taking breaks or engaging in activities that bring us joy, our stress levels soar, and we become more susceptible to burnout. By incorporating self-care practices such as yoga into our daily routine, we give ourselves permission to rest, rejuvenate, and restore our energy, enabling us to better cope with the demands of life.

Moreover, self-care plays a vital role in improving our mental and emotional well-being. Engaging in activities that bring us happiness and fulfillment boosts our mood, reduces anxiety, and enhances our overall mental health. Yoga, in particular, has been shown to increase the production of feel-good hormones such as endorphins, promoting a sense of well-being and reducing stress-induced symptoms like irritability and mood swings.

In conclusion, self-care is essential for stress reduction, and yoga serves as a powerful tool to achieve this goal. By prioritizing self-care, we give ourselves permission to nurture our mind, body, and soul, resulting in reduced stress levels and increased serenity. So, whether you are a seasoned yogi or just starting your journey, don't forget to take time for yourself and embrace the importance of self-care in finding peace in a chaotic world.

Nurturing Healthy Relationships and Boundaries

In our fast-paced and chaotic world, finding serenity can seem like an elusive goal. However, incorporating yoga into our lives can provide a much-needed respite from the stress and help us build healthier relationships and boundaries. This subchapter explores the powerful connection between yoga and nurturing healthy relationships, offering practical insights and techniques for anyone seeking to create more harmonious connections in their lives.

Yoga is not just about physical postures; it is a holistic practice that encompasses the mind, body, and spirit. By focusing on breath control, meditation, and mindfulness, yoga teaches us to be present in the moment and cultivate self-awareness. This self-awareness is the foundation for nurturing healthy relationships with ourselves and others.

When we practice yoga, we learn to listen to our bodies and honor our limits. This principle translates into our relationships as well. By setting boundaries and understanding our own needs, we can establish healthier dynamics with those around us. Yoga encourages us to prioritize self-care and recognize when we need time alone or space to recharge. By communicating our boundaries effectively, we create an environment where healthy and respectful relationships can thrive.

Furthermore, yoga teaches us compassion and empathy, essential qualities for building strong connections. As we cultivate self-compassion on the mat, we learn to extend it to others. By practicing non-judgment and embracing diversity, we foster inclusivity and understanding in our relationships. Yoga helps us develop the ability to truly listen and support others, creating an environment where everyone feels heard and valued.

The subchapter also delves into the importance of communication in nurturing healthy relationships. Yoga emphasizes the power of mindful communication, teaching us to speak from a place of kindness and authenticity. By practicing active listening and expressing ourselves with clarity and compassion, we can resolve conflicts and strengthen our bonds.

In conclusion, yoga is a powerful tool for nurturing healthy relationships and establishing boundaries. By incorporating yoga into our lives, we develop self-awareness, compassion, and effective communication skills, all of which are crucial for building harmonious connections. Whether you are new to yoga or a seasoned practitioner, the insights and techniques shared in this subchapter will empower you to cultivate healthier relationships and find serenity in our chaotic world.

Finding Balance in Work, Rest, and Play

In our fast-paced and chaotic world, finding balance is essential for our overall well-being. The demands of work, family, and personal life can often leave us feeling overwhelmed and stressed. It is in times like these that incorporating yoga into our daily routine can provide the perfect antidote. Yoga for Stress Relief: Finding Serenity in a Chaotic World offers valuable insights on how to strike a harmonious balance between work, rest, and play.

Work, rest, and play are three essential components of a fulfilling life, and finding equilibrium among them is crucial. Many of us tend to prioritize work above everything else, often neglecting our need for rest and play. However, this unbalanced approach can lead to burnout, decreased productivity, and a diminished quality of life.

Yoga teaches us the importance of finding harmony in all aspects of our lives. Through the practice of asanas, pranayama, and meditation, we learn to cultivate mindfulness and become more attuned to our body, mind, and spirit. This awareness enables us to identify when we are out of balance and make the necessary adjustments to restore equilibrium.

The subchapter "Finding Balance in Work, Rest, and Play" delves deeper into the significance of each of these three elements and provides practical tips on how to achieve a healthy balance. It emphasizes the importance of setting boundaries and prioritizing self-care to avoid burnout. The subchapter also explores the transformative power of rest and play, highlighting how these activities can rejuvenate our mind and body, boosting our overall well-being.

Moreover, this subchapter includes a variety of yoga poses, breathing exercises, and mindfulness techniques specifically curated to support work-life balance. These practices can be easily incorporated into our daily routine, helping us to release stress, improve focus, and enhance our overall sense of calm.

Whether you are a yoga enthusiast or completely new to the practice, Yoga for Stress Relief: Finding Serenity in a Chaotic World offers valuable insights and practical guidance to help you find balance in work, rest, and play. By embracing the principles of yoga, you can transform your life, find serenity amidst chaos, and create a harmonious existence that nurtures your mind, body, and spirit.

Chapter 6: Yoga for Specific Stress-Related Conditions

Yoga for Anxiety and Panic Disorders

In today's chaotic world, stress and anxiety have become common companions in many people's lives. The constant pressures of work, relationships, and societal expectations can often leave us feeling overwhelmed and on edge. However, there is a powerful tool that can help us find serenity amidst the chaos – yoga.

Yoga is not just a physical practice; it is a holistic approach to well-being that combines physical postures, breath control, meditation, and mindfulness. When it comes to anxiety and panic disorders, yoga can be a game-changer. Its gentle, yet powerful techniques can help calm the mind, relax the body, and bring about a sense of inner peace.

One of the key elements of yoga for anxiety and panic disorders is the focus on deep, conscious breathing. Shallow breathing is a common symptom of anxiety, and it only serves to perpetuate the cycle of panic. By practicing deep, diaphragmatic breathing, we can activate the body's relaxation response and bring about a sense of calmness and control.

Another important aspect of yoga for anxiety is the physical postures, known as asanas. These postures help release tension from the body, stretch and strengthen muscles, and improve overall flexibility. Specific poses like the Child's Pose, Standing

Forward Bend, and Corpse Pose can be particularly beneficial in reducing anxiety and promoting relaxation.

In addition to breath control and physical postures, meditation and mindfulness play a crucial role in managing anxiety and panic disorders. By quieting the mind and focusing on the present moment, we can break free from the constant stream of worries and fears that contribute to our anxiety. Regular practice of meditation and mindfulness can help rewire the brain, making us more resilient to stress and anxiety triggers.

It is important to note that yoga is not a quick fix for anxiety and panic disorders. It is a journey that requires dedication, patience, and consistency. However, with regular practice, yoga can become a powerful tool in our arsenal against anxiety. It can provide us with a sense of empowerment, allowing us to take control of our mental and emotional well-being.

If you are struggling with anxiety or panic disorders, incorporating yoga into your daily routine can be a transformative experience. Seek out qualified yoga instructors or online resources that specialize in yoga for anxiety. Remember, everyone's journey is unique, so find what works best for you. Give yourself permission to slow down, breathe, and find serenity amidst the chaos through the practice of yoga.

Yoga for Depression and Mood Disorders

In today's fast-paced and chaotic world, it is not uncommon for individuals to experience stress, anxiety, and even depression. Fortunately, yoga offers a holistic approach to addressing these mental health concerns. By combining physical postures, breathing exercises, and meditation, yoga can help individuals find serenity and relief from the symptoms of depression and mood disorders.

Depression is a serious mental health condition that affects millions of people worldwide. It can lead to a persistent feeling of sadness, loss of interest in activities, and a lack of energy. Yoga can be a valuable tool in managing depression as it helps to release tension, improve blood flow, and activate the body's relaxation response.

One of the key components of yoga for depression is the practice of asanas, or physical postures. These postures help to stretch and strengthen the body, releasing built-up tension and promoting a sense of well-being. Certain poses, such as the downward-facing dog and the warrior pose, can help to energize the body and uplift the mood.

Breathing exercises, or pranayama, are another integral part of yoga for depression. Deep, slow breathing techniques can activate the parasympathetic nervous system, which promotes relaxation and reduces stress. By focusing on the breath, individuals can calm their minds and find a sense of peace and tranquility.

Meditation is a powerful tool for managing depression and mood disorders. By practicing mindfulness and being present in the moment, individuals can cultivate a sense of inner peace and acceptance. Meditation helps to quiet the mind, reduce negative thoughts, and improve overall mental well-being.

Yoga also encourages self-care and self-compassion, which are crucial for managing depression. Practicing yoga allows individuals to connect with their bodies, listen to their needs, and offer themselves kindness and understanding. This self-nurturing aspect of yoga can help individuals develop a positive relationship with themselves and cultivate a sense of self-worth.

If you are struggling with depression or a mood disorder, incorporating yoga into your daily routine can be immensely beneficial. However, it is important to remember that yoga is not a substitute for professional help. If you are experiencing severe depression or if your symptoms worsen, it is essential to seek support from a qualified healthcare professional.

In conclusion, yoga offers a holistic approach to managing depression and mood disorders. By combining physical postures, breathing exercises, and meditation, yoga helps individuals find serenity in a chaotic world. Whether you are new to yoga or an experienced practitioner, incorporating yoga into your life can support your mental well-being and help you find relief from the challenges of depression.

Yoga for Insomnia and Sleep Disorders

In our fast-paced and chaotic world, getting a good night's sleep has become increasingly difficult. Insomnia and sleep disorders have become all too common, leaving many individuals feeling tired, irritable, and unable to function at their best. If you're struggling with sleepless nights, yoga may hold the key to finding serenity and restoring balance to your life.

Yoga is an ancient practice that combines physical postures, breathing exercises, and meditation to promote overall well-being. It has been proven to reduce stress, anxiety, and depression, making it an effective tool for managing sleep-related issues. By incorporating a regular yoga routine into your life, you can create a calming bedtime ritual that will help you unwind and prepare your mind and body for a restful night's sleep.

One of the primary benefits of yoga for insomnia and sleep disorders is its ability to activate the parasympathetic nervous system, also known as the "rest and digest" response. Through gentle movement and deep breathing, yoga triggers a relaxation response in the body, promoting a sense of calm and reducing the release of stress hormones.

Certain yoga poses are particularly beneficial for promoting sleep. Forward folds, such as Uttanasana (Standing Forward Bend) or Paschimottanasana (Seated Forward Bend), help to calm the mind and release tension from the body. Gentle inversions, such as Viparita Karani (Legs-Up-The-Wall Pose), can also be effective in promoting relaxation and improving blood circulation.

In addition to physical postures, incorporating pranayama, or breath control, into your yoga practice can be highly beneficial for sleep. Deep breathing exercises, such as Nadi Shodhana (Alternate Nostril Breathing), can help to balance the nervous system, alleviate anxiety, and induce a state of deep relaxation.

Meditation and mindfulness practices are also integral components of yoga that can aid in overcoming insomnia and sleep disorders. By focusing your attention on the present moment and cultivating a sense of inner peace, you can quiet your racing thoughts and create an environment conducive to sleep.

Remember, it's essential to approach your yoga practice with patience and consistency. While the benefits of yoga for sleep may not be immediate, with time and practice, you will gradually notice improvements in the quality and duration of your sleep.

So, if you find yourself tossing and turning night after night, consider incorporating yoga into your daily routine. By embracing this ancient practice, you can find serenity in a chaotic world and experience the restorative power of a good night's sleep.

Chapter 7: Yoga and Beyond: Integrating Other Stress-Relieving Practices

Ayurveda: The Sister Science of Yoga for Holistic Healing

In the quest for finding serenity in a chaotic world, many individuals turn to yoga as a means of finding peace and balance. However, what most people are unaware of is that yoga has a sister science known as Ayurveda, which complements and enhances the benefits of yoga for holistic healing.

Ayurveda, derived from the Sanskrit words "ayur" (life) and "veda" (knowledge), is an ancient Indian system of medicine that focuses on achieving optimal health and wellness. It is based on the belief that the mind, body, and spirit are interconnected, and the key to good health lies in balancing these elements.

Just like yoga, Ayurveda seeks to promote well-being through various practices and principles. It emphasizes the importance of a healthy lifestyle, proper nutrition, herbal remedies, and mindful living. By incorporating Ayurvedic principles into your yoga practice, you can experience a deeper level of healing and transformation.

One of the fundamental principles of Ayurveda is the concept of doshas, which are three biological energies that govern our physical and mental well-being. These doshas, known as Vata, Pitta, and Kapha, determine our unique constitution and influence our physical characteristics, temperament, and susceptibility to certain ailments. By understanding your dosha type, you can tailor your yoga practice and lifestyle choices to achieve balance and harmony.

For example, if you have a Vata constitution, characterized by traits such as creativity and flexibility but prone to anxiety and restlessness, you may benefit from grounding and calming yoga practices. On the other hand, individuals with a Pitta constitution, characterized by ambition and intensity but prone to irritability and inflammation, may find relief through cooling and balancing yoga poses.

Ayurveda also offers a wealth of herbal remedies and dietary guidelines to support your yoga practice and overall well-being. By incorporating Ayurvedic herbs, such as ashwagandha for stress relief or turmeric for inflammation, into your daily routine, you can enhance the healing effects of yoga and promote a state of holistic wellness.

In conclusion, Ayurveda and yoga are inseparable sisters on the path to holistic healing. By integrating Ayurvedic principles into your yoga practice, you can attain a deeper level of self-awareness, balance your doshas, and unlock the true potential of your mind, body, and spirit. Embracing this ancient wisdom can lead you to find serenity in a chaotic world and experience lasting well-being.

Nutrition and Diet for Stress Reduction

In today's fast-paced and chaotic world, stress has become an inevitable part of our everyday lives. From work pressures to personal challenges, stress takes a toll on both our physical and mental well-being. However, by incorporating certain dietary changes and focusing on nutrition, we can effectively reduce stress levels and find serenity amidst the chaos. This subchapter discusses the importance of nutrition and diet for stress reduction, specifically within the context of yoga.

Yoga, a holistic practice that combines physical postures, breathing exercises, and meditation, has long been recognized for its stress-reducing benefits. While yoga helps to calm the mind and relax the body, the role of nutrition cannot be overlooked in this journey towards stress relief.

When it comes to combating stress through nutrition, it is essential to focus on nourishing our bodies with the right foods. A well-balanced diet rich in vitamins, minerals, and antioxidants can provide the necessary support to our nervous system and help combat the negative effects of stress. Incorporating whole foods, such as fruits, vegetables, whole grains, and lean proteins, is key to promoting overall well-being and reducing stress levels.

Certain nutrients have been found to have a direct impact on stress reduction. For instance, foods rich in B vitamins, such as leafy greens, legumes, and whole grains, play a crucial role in supporting the nervous system and maintaining energy levels. Omega-3 fatty acids, found in fatty fish, flaxseeds, and walnuts, have been shown to reduce inflammation and promote a sense of calmness. Additionally, magnesium, present in foods like spinach, almonds, and avocados, helps relax muscles and promote better sleep, ultimately reducing stress.

In contrast, it is important to limit or avoid foods that can exacerbate stress. Caffeine, found in coffee, tea, and energy drinks, can increase anxiety and disrupt sleep patterns. Similarly, refined sugars and processed foods can lead to energy crashes and mood swings, intensifying stress levels. By making conscious choices and opting for healthier alternatives, we can better support our bodies and manage stress effectively.

In conclusion, nutrition and diet play an integral role in reducing stress levels, particularly when combined with the practice of yoga. By nourishing our bodies with wholesome foods and avoiding stress-inducing substances, we can promote a sense of calmness and well-being within ourselves. Remember, finding serenity in a chaotic world begins with taking care of our physical and mental health.

Exploring Other Complementary Therapies for Stress Relief

In addition to practicing yoga, there are several other complementary therapies that can greatly contribute to stress relief and help us find serenity in a chaotic world. These therapies work in harmony with yoga and can provide an extra boost to our overall well-being. In this subchapter, we will explore some of these alternative therapies and discuss how they can enhance our stress management techniques.

One such complementary therapy is aromatherapy. The use of essential oils derived from plants has been known to have a profound impact on our emotions and mental state. Certain scents, such as lavender, chamomile, and bergamot, have calming properties that can promote relaxation and reduce stress levels. Incorporating aromatherapy into your yoga practice by diffusing essential oils or using them in massage oils can create a soothing and tranquil environment, intensifying the stress-relieving effects of yoga.

Another effective complementary therapy is acupuncture. Originating from ancient Chinese medicine, acupuncture involves the insertion of thin needles into specific points on the body to stimulate energy flow and restore balance. This practice has been found to reduce stress and anxiety by activating the body's natural healing response. Combining acupuncture with yoga can enhance the benefits of both practices, allowing for a deeper sense of relaxation and stress relief.

Massage therapy is yet another complementary therapy that pairs well with yoga. The physical manipulation of muscles through massage can release tension and promote relaxation. Practicing yoga can help increase body awareness, making massage therapy more effective in relieving stress-related muscle tension and promoting overall well-being.

Furthermore, meditation, although often incorporated into yoga practice, can also be explored as a standalone complementary therapy. Regular meditation practice can calm the mind, reduce anxiety, and improve focus. It complements yoga by helping to cultivate a sense of inner peace and serenity.

By exploring these complementary therapies alongside your yoga practice, you can create a comprehensive stress relief routine that addresses both the physical and mental aspects of stress. Each therapy offers unique benefits that, when combined with yoga, can help you find serenity amidst the chaos of everyday life. Experiment with different techniques to discover which combination works best for you, and embrace the journey towards a more balanced and stress-free existence.

Chapter 8: Overcoming Challenges and Maintaining Motivation

Overcoming Resistance to Change and Establishing a Routine

Change is an inevitable part of life, and yet many of us find ourselves resisting it. Whether it's a new job, a new relationship, or even a new yoga practice, we often feel a sense of discomfort and fear when faced with something unfamiliar. However, it is through embracing change that we can truly grow and find serenity in a chaotic world.

In the world of yoga, resistance to change can manifest in various ways. It might be the resistance to trying a new pose, attending a different class, or even embarking on a yoga retreat. We may find ourselves clinging to the familiar, afraid to step out of our comfort zone. But by overcoming this resistance, we open ourselves up to new possibilities and experiences.

One effective way to overcome resistance to change is by establishing a routine. Creating a consistent yoga practice can provide a sense of stability and structure amidst the chaos of life. By committing to a regular practice, we cultivate discipline and develop a deep connection with ourselves and our bodies.

Establishing a routine can also help us overcome the fear of the unknown. When we know what to expect, we feel more confident and at ease. Start by setting aside a specific time each day for your yoga practice. It could be early in the morning, during your lunch break, or in the evening before bed. Find a time that works best for you and stick to it.

In addition to a consistent practice time, create a dedicated space for your yoga practice. It could be a corner of your living room, a spare bedroom, or even a small outdoor area. Fill this space with items that inspire and motivate you, such as candles, incense, or meaningful objects. Having a designated space will help you establish a sense of sacredness and focus during your practice.

As you embark on your yoga journey, remember to be patient and kind to yourself. Change takes time, and it's normal to experience setbacks along the way. Embrace the challenges and view them as opportunities for growth. With persistence and determination, you will overcome resistance to change and find serenity in the chaos.

So, take that first step towards change by establishing a routine and embracing the unknown. Your yoga practice will become a sanctuary, a place where you can find solace and relief from the stresses of everyday life. Embrace the journey, and let yoga guide you towards serenity in a chaotic world.

Dealing with Setbacks and Managing Expectations

In the journey of life, setbacks are inevitable. Whether it's a personal challenge, a professional setback, or even a hurdle in your yoga practice, setbacks can leave us feeling discouraged and overwhelmed. However, learning how to deal with setbacks and managing our expectations can be the key to finding serenity in a chaotic world.

Yoga, a practice that combines physical postures, breathwork, and meditation, offers valuable insights and tools for managing setbacks. When faced with adversity, yoga teaches us to approach it with mindfulness, compassion, and resilience. It encourages us to embrace the present moment and find peace within ourselves, even when the world around us feels chaotic.

One of the first steps in dealing with setbacks is acknowledging and accepting that they are a natural part of life. By understanding that setbacks are temporary and often necessary for growth, we can shift our perspective and approach them with a sense of curiosity rather than frustration. Yoga teaches us to breathe through challenges and observe our reactions without judgment, allowing us to cultivate a more balanced mindset.

Managing expectations is another crucial aspect of dealing with setbacks. Often, we set unrealistic expectations for ourselves, leading to disappointment and self-criticism when things don't go as planned. Yoga encourages us to let go of perfectionism and embrace our journey as it unfolds. By focusing on the process rather than the outcome, we can find joy in the present moment and appreciate the progress we make, no matter how small it may seem.

Practicing yoga regularly can also help us build resilience and bounce back from setbacks more efficiently. The physical postures, or asanas, challenge our bodies and minds, teaching us to find stability and balance even in challenging situations. Through breathwork and meditation, we learn to quiet the mind, reduce stress, and cultivate a sense of inner calm. These tools can be invaluable when facing setbacks, helping us navigate through difficult times with grace and resilience.

Ultimately, dealing with setbacks and managing expectations is an ongoing practice. By incorporating the principles of yoga into our lives, we can develop a deeper understanding of ourselves and the world around us. Through self-reflection, self-compassion, and a commitment to growth, we can find serenity amidst the chaos and emerge stronger from any setback that comes our way.

Whether you're new to yoga or a seasoned practitioner, embracing these teachings can help you navigate the ups and downs of life with more ease and grace. So, take a deep breath, roll out your mat, and embark on a journey of self-discovery, resilience, and stress relief through the transformative power of yoga.

Cultivating Mindfulness and Gratitude for Long-Term Well-Being

In today's fast-paced and chaotic world, finding serenity and inner peace can seem like an impossible task. Stress and anxiety have become a common part of our daily lives, affecting our overall well-being. Thankfully, there is a powerful tool that can help us navigate through the challenges and find solace – yoga.

Yoga is not just a physical exercise; it is a holistic practice that combines movement, breath, and mindfulness to create a harmonious mind-body connection. By incorporating yoga into our lives, we can cultivate mindfulness and gratitude, leading to long-term well-being.

Mindfulness is the art of being fully present and aware of the present moment without judgment. In yoga, this is achieved through various techniques such as breath awareness and conscious movement. By practicing mindfulness on the mat, we learn to bring this awareness into our daily lives, allowing us to be fully present in every moment.

Gratitude is another powerful tool that can transform our lives. When we cultivate gratitude, we shift our focus from what is lacking to what we already have. Yoga provides us with an opportunity to express gratitude for our bodies, our breath, and the simple pleasures of life. By practicing gratitude, we develop a positive mindset, which in turn enhances our overall well-being.

Cultivating mindfulness and gratitude through yoga requires consistent practice and dedication. It is not a quick fix but rather a lifelong journey. However, the benefits are immense. Regular yoga practice can reduce stress, anxiety, and depression, improve sleep quality, increase self-awareness, and enhance overall physical and mental health.

To incorporate mindfulness and gratitude into your yoga practice, start by setting an intention for each session. This can be as simple as expressing gratitude for the opportunity to practice or setting an intention to be present and mindful on the mat. Throughout your practice, focus on your breath, allowing it to anchor you in the present moment.

As you move through the poses, pay attention to your body without judgment. Notice any sensations, thoughts, or emotions that arise, and simply observe them without getting attached. This practice of non-judgmental awareness can help you develop a more compassionate and accepting attitude towards yourself and others.

After your practice, take a few moments to reflect on what you are grateful for. It can be something as small as the warmth of the sun or the support of loved ones. By ending your practice with gratitude, you carry this positive energy into the rest of your day.

In conclusion, cultivating mindfulness and gratitude through yoga is a powerful way to find serenity in a chaotic world. By incorporating these practices into our lives, we can enhance our overall well-being and create a positive mindset. Whether you are a beginner or an experienced yogi, embracing mindfulness and gratitude will transform your yoga practice and your life. Start today and experience the profound benefits for yourself.

Chapter 9: The Power of Community and Support

Joining Yoga Classes and Finding Like-Minded Individuals

One of the most rewarding aspects of practicing yoga is the opportunity to connect with like-minded individuals who share a common interest in personal growth, health, and self-discovery. Yoga classes provide a perfect platform for individuals to come together, support one another, and create a sense of community. Whether you are a beginner or an experienced yogi, joining a yoga class can greatly enhance your practice and help you find serenity in a chaotic world.

When you join a yoga class, you not only benefit from the guidance of a knowledgeable instructor but also surround yourself with a diverse group of individuals who are on a similar journey of self-improvement. This community of like-minded individuals can provide a sense of belonging and support, making your yoga practice even more enriching.

Finding a yoga class that resonates with you is essential. Look for a studio or instructor that aligns with your values, teaching style preferences, and level of experience. Many studios offer a variety of classes, including beginner, intermediate, and advanced levels, as well as specialized classes such as prenatal yoga or restorative yoga. Take the time to explore different options and find the class that suits your needs and goals.

Once you have found the right yoga class, be open to connecting with your fellow practitioners. Engage in conversations before or after class, ask questions, and share your experiences. You may be surprised by the wisdom and insights you gain from others who are on a similar path.

Joining a yoga class also provides an opportunity to learn from experienced instructors who can guide you in refining your practice. They can offer modifications and adjustments specific to your body and help you deepen your understanding of the poses and breathing techniques. Through regular attendance and commitment, you will witness the progress you make and feel motivated to continue your yoga journey.

Remember, yoga is not just about the physical practice; it is a holistic approach to well-being. By joining a yoga class and connecting with like-minded individuals, you are not only improving your physical health but also nurturing your mental and emotional well-being.

In conclusion, joining a yoga class is a powerful way to enhance your practice and find serenity in a chaotic world. Embrace the opportunity to connect with like-minded individuals, learn from experienced instructors, and create a sense of community. Through yoga, you will not only find stress relief but also discover a path to personal growth, self-acceptance, and a deeper understanding of yourself and the world around you.

Building a Support Network for Stress Relief

In our fast-paced and chaotic world, stress has become an inevitable part of our lives. The constant pressure to meet deadlines, juggle responsibilities, and maintain a work-life balance can leave us feeling overwhelmed and exhausted. However, there are ways to find serenity amidst this chaos, and one effective method is through building a support network for stress relief, with yoga at its core.

Yoga is not just a physical exercise; it is a holistic practice that combines movement, breath control, and meditation. It has been proven to reduce stress by promoting relaxation and improving overall well-being. But practicing yoga alone is not enough to combat stress; having a support network can make all the difference.

Your support network can include friends, family, and even fellow yogis who understand and empathize with your stressors. Here are a few tips to help you build a strong support network for stress relief:

1. Find a yoga studio or community center near you: Joining a yoga class or group can introduce you to like-minded individuals who are also seeking stress relief. Sharing your experiences and challenges with others who understand can provide a sense of belonging and support.

2. Attend yoga workshops or retreats: These events offer a unique opportunity to connect with people who share your passion for yoga. Participating in workshops or retreats allows you to deepen

your practice while forming meaningful connections with others who can become part of your support network.

3. Utilize online platforms: In this digital age, there are numerous online communities and forums dedicated to yoga and stress relief. Engaging with these platforms can help you connect with individuals from all over the world, creating a diverse and supportive network.

4. Seek professional guidance: Consider working with a yoga instructor or therapist who specializes in stress management. They can provide personalized guidance and support, helping you navigate the challenges of stress in a healthy and effective manner.

Remember, building a support network takes time and effort. Be open to forming new connections, nurturing existing relationships, and seeking support when needed. Your support network will not only provide you with encouragement and understanding but also offer valuable insights and techniques for managing stress.

In conclusion, yoga is a powerful tool for stress relief, but it is even more effective when practiced within a supportive community. By building a support network that includes fellow yogis, friends, and professionals, you can find solace, inspiration, and guidance on your journey towards serenity in a chaotic world.

Sharing Your Journey and Inspiring Others

In the fast-paced and chaotic world we live in, finding serenity and peace of mind can often feel like an elusive goal. However, through the practice of yoga, we can tap into our inner calm and experience true stress relief. But what if we could take it a step further? What if we could not only find serenity for ourselves but also inspire others to do the same? This subchapter explores the power of sharing your journey and inspiring others in the realm of yoga.

Yoga, at its core, is a deeply personal practice. It allows us to connect with our bodies, minds, and spirits in a way that is unique to each individual. However, this personal journey doesn't have to be a solitary one. By sharing our experiences, struggles, and triumphs, we have the potential to create a community of support and encouragement.

Sharing your yoga journey with others can take many forms. It could be as simple as discussing your practice with friends and family or sharing photos and updates on social media. You might choose to start a blog or write articles for yoga publications, documenting your progress and offering insights along the way. You could even consider becoming a yoga teacher, guiding others on their own paths of self-discovery and stress relief.

The act of sharing your journey is not only beneficial for others but also for yourself. It reinforces your commitment and dedication to the practice, as well as deepens your understanding of the principles and benefits of yoga. By articulating your experiences, you gain a greater sense of clarity and insight into your own journey.

Inspiring others through your yoga journey is a powerful way to give back to the community. Through your words and actions, you have the ability to motivate and encourage others to embark on their own path towards serenity and stress relief. Your journey serves as a beacon of hope, showing others that it is possible to find peace in a chaotic world.

Remember, however, that inspiring others does not mean projecting an image of perfection. It's important to be authentic and transparent about your own challenges and setbacks. By sharing your vulnerabilities, you create a safe space for others to explore their own journeys without fear of judgment or failure.

Conclusion,

sharing your yoga journey and inspiring others is a beautiful and transformative way to contribute to the yoga community. Whether it's through conversations, writing, or teaching, the impact you can have on others is immeasurable. So, embrace the power of sharing, and let your journey be a guiding light for those seeking serenity in a chaotic world.

Chapter 10: Embracing Serenity in a Chaotic World

Embracing Imperfections and Letting Go of Control

In our fast-paced and chaotic world, it is easy to get caught up in the pursuit of perfection and control. We strive to have the perfect body, the perfect career, and the perfect life. However, this constant need for control often leads to stress, anxiety, and a sense of dissatisfaction.

Yoga teaches us the importance of embracing imperfections and letting go of control. It encourages us to accept ourselves as we are, with all our flaws and limitations. Instead of striving for perfection, yoga invites us to find peace and contentment in the present moment.

One of the fundamental principles of yoga is the concept of non-attachment. This means letting go of the need to control every aspect of our lives and instead surrendering to the flow of life. Through the practice of yoga, we learn to release our grip on the external world and focus on the internal sensations of our bodies and minds.

By embracing imperfections, we create space for growth and self-acceptance. Yoga teaches us that imperfections are not something to be ashamed of, but rather opportunities for growth and self-discovery. When we let go of the need for control, we can embrace our imperfections and learn from them.

In yoga, we learn to cultivate self-compassion and kindness towards ourselves. Instead of criticizing ourselves for not being perfect, we learn to be gentle and loving towards ourselves. We recognize that we are human beings, and it is natural to make mistakes and have limitations.

Through the practice of yoga, we develop a sense of surrender and trust in the process of life. We let go of the need to control every outcome and instead trust that everything is unfolding exactly as it should. This trust allows us to find serenity and peace in the midst of chaos.

So, whether you are a seasoned yogi or just starting your yoga journey, embracing imperfections and letting go of control is a crucial lesson to learn. By practicing yoga, you can find serenity in a chaotic world and cultivate a deep sense of self-acceptance and peace. Embrace imperfections, let go of control, and discover the beauty of surrendering to the present moment.

Cultivating Inner Peace and Serenity Through Yoga

In today's fast-paced and chaotic world, finding inner peace and serenity can often feel like an elusive pursuit. The demands of work, family, and societal expectations can leave us feeling overwhelmed, stressed, and disconnected from ourselves. However, there is a powerful tool that can help us navigate through the challenges of life and find a sense of calm amidst the chaos – yoga.

Yoga is not just a physical exercise; it is a holistic practice that combines breath control, meditation, and a series of postures to harmonize the mind, body, and spirit. By incorporating yoga into our daily routine, we can create a space within ourselves that is free from anxiety, stress, and negativity.

One of the primary benefits of yoga is its ability to activate the relaxation response in our bodies. When we practice deep breathing and mindful movement, our nervous system shifts from the fight-or-flight response to the rest-and-digest mode. This physiological shift helps to reduce stress hormones, lower blood pressure, and promote a sense of calmness and well-being.

Moreover, yoga teaches us to be present in the moment and cultivate self-awareness. Through regular practice, we learn to observe our thoughts without judgment and let go of negative emotions that no longer serve us. This process of self-reflection allows us to develop a deeper understanding of ourselves, leading to increased self-acceptance and inner peace.

In addition to its mental and emotional benefits, yoga also provides numerous physical advantages. Regular practice improves flexibility, strength, and balance, thereby enhancing overall physical well-being. It can also help alleviate conditions such as chronic pain, insomnia, and fatigue, which are often associated with stress.

To cultivate inner peace and serenity through yoga, it is essential to establish a consistent practice. Start by dedicating a few minutes each day to focus on your breath and perform simple yoga postures. As you become more comfortable, gradually increase the duration and complexity of your practice. Consider joining a yoga class or seeking guidance from a certified instructor to ensure proper alignment and maximize the benefits.

Remember, yoga is a personal journey, and each individual's experience will be unique. Embrace the process and be patient with yourself. With time and dedication, you will discover the transformative power of yoga, finding serenity and balance in all aspects of your life.

Living a Balanced and Stress-Free Life in a Chaotic World

In today's fast-paced and chaotic world, finding serenity and achieving a balanced life may seem like an impossible task. However, through the practice of yoga, we can discover ways to navigate the stresses and challenges of daily life and cultivate a sense of peace and tranquillity.

Yoga is not just about physical exercise; it is a holistic approach to wellbeing that encompasses the mind, body, and spirit. By incorporating yoga into our daily routine, we can cultivate mindfulness, reduce stress, and find balance amidst the chaos.

One of the key principles of yoga is the importance of breath. The breath is a powerful tool that can help us navigate stress and restore equilibrium. Through deep and intentional breathing, we activate the parasympathetic nervous system, which promotes relaxation and reduces the production of stress hormones. By incorporating breathwork techniques into our yoga practice, such as alternate nostril breathing or deep belly breathing, we can instantly create a sense of calm and balance within ourselves.

Another essential aspect of living a balanced and stress-free life is the practice of mindfulness. Mindfulness involves being fully present in the moment, without judgment or attachment to thoughts or emotions. By practicing mindfulness during our yoga practice, we can train our minds to let go of worries and anxieties, and instead focus on the present moment. This allows us to experience a sense of peace and clarity, even in the midst of chaos.

In addition to breathwork and mindfulness, yoga also offers physical postures, known as asanas, that help release tension and promote relaxation. Through regular practice, we can strengthen our bodies, increase flexibility, and release stored stress and tension. By incorporating poses such as forward folds, gentle twists, and restorative poses into our yoga practice, we can create a sense of balance and serenity in our bodies.

Ultimately, living a balanced and stress-free life in a chaotic world is about finding harmony within ourselves. Yoga provides us with the tools and practices we need to navigate the challenges of daily life with grace and ease. By incorporating breathwork, mindfulness, and physical postures into our yoga practice, we can cultivate a sense of serenity and balance that transcends the chaos around us. So, start your journey towards a more peaceful and harmonious life today and discover the transformative power of yoga.